Intermittent Fasting Done The Right Way:

Step by step guide on how to properly Fast and regain your health

By Terry James

Table of Contents

Introduction

What is Intermittent Fasting (IF)?

The word "Intermittent" is defined as "occurring in irregular intervals". The word fasting is an act in which one refrains from a certain activity for a specific period of time. Simply put Intermittent Fasting is refraining from food for a certain time period. IF has two components

- A fasting period: time interval in which you refrain from eating

- A feeding window: time interval in which you are allowed to eat.

What If Intermittent Fasting (IF) is not?

- IF is not a magic bullet for weight loss, you will not lose 10lbs in one week. You may however make consistent loss such as 1pound per week.

- IF does not claim to be the best diet or the best approach to dieting for everyone. IF is a simplified diet method that works best for the busy individual.

- IF is not a necessity. IF, like every other diet is just a tool to help you lose weight. Think of it as another tool to add to your toolbox for fat-loss. There are plenty of other ways to lose weight.

Why should you fast?

Intermittent fasting has many benefits, here are a few.

- Lower blood pressure

- Lower oxidative stress

- Increased fat burning

- Increased metabolic rate during the fast

- Improved appetite control

- Improved blood sugar control

- Improved cardiovascular function

Who is this manual for?

This manual is for those who

- Want to learn the basic of intermittent fasting

- Want a to improve their health

- Experience a consistent and manageable way to lose weight.

- Want to adhere to a diet and without the hassle of being limited to certain foods.

- This manual assumes that you have an exercise program to accompany an IF diet program.

Maximum fat loss cannot be achieved through diet alone instead Fasting. it is a combination of exercise and diet that produces maximum fat loss. If you do not have an exercise program do not fright. An exercise program can be as simply as jogging for 30minutes a day. However it should be noted that a well- designed training program that is tailored towards your goal will produce the best results.

How Intermittent Fasting Works

Intermittent fasting is a controlled pattern of fasting that is made in an alternate way. Fasting? Meaning "not eat"? Yes, I really mean not to eat. Most of us when we are hungry, we chow down on foods that we can grab. This includes junk foods, processed foods and most of the time, fast foods. Anywhere we go, we see fast foods. Anywhere we go, we see street foods and so on. We eat three meals in a day and for most of us, three meals are not yet enough. We tend to feed ourselves more every time we feel the hunger or every time we feel the crave for food. We know very much that this is wrong but we do not think of it and push ourselves to give in to that craving. Regular meals are only breakfast, lunch and dinner. These are the only meals that are important to us. Every other meal is just additional and most of the time not needed which causes us to add our weight and produce fat. When we do not work too much and physical activity is done most of the time then we might as well feed ourselves of hunger. But if we do not do physical activity much, then we should not give in to this temptous craving.

So what do we do?

This is where I can introduce intermittent fasting. This is when we eat our daily meals in a day and do fasting for the next twenty four hours. We do not necessarily mean that you cannot take in anything in your stomach.

We just want you take in water or any healthy drink including fruit juice. But we recommend that water is better.

Water does a lot of good things in our body. It cleans our body and helps flush out unhealthy food. There are a lot of scientific studies and researches that proves that intermittent fasting is very beneficial to our health. Remember before that our ancestors did not have any fast foods, junk foods or street foods whenever they are hungry. What do they do? They drink water in order for their hunger to be lost. Most of the time, we feel hunger not because we really are hungry but our body and mind just dictates us to eat because it is used to. We call this mental hunger. Sometimes, our minds just cheat us.

So this is the tip on intermittent fasting. Example, today you can eat as much food as you like. But be prepared that after dinner tonight you are just allowed to drink water afterwards for twenty four hours. Drink water as much as you need to feed your hunger. This process will train your body and mind to not let you eat when you do not need to eat. This fasting will eventually lead your body to use the stored fat and energy that has not been used for a long period of time. So you will lose weight and keep you healthier. Intermittent fasting is not advisable for all people. This is only good for individuals without health problems. Whenever you wanted to try Intermittent fasting, you should consult first with your doctor before

you push through.

Chapter One

Basic Dietary Guidelines

Will Intermittent Fasting Help You Lose Weight

Under certain circumstances, there is a great deal of evidence that says intermittent fasting can help with burning fat. Intermittent fasting is spacing your last meal of the day and your first meal the next day farther apart to as much as 16 hours. The rational is that after you eat, your body takes about six to eight hours to metabolize that glycogen, then to continue functioning it goes into your fat stores. But if we start feeding our body before that six to eight time period, or before the glycogen has been used, we never allow our system to tap into our fat storage. This makes it very difficult to ever lose weight. Of course we can go too far when we fast. When we go past a certain point, our system realizes it isn't going to get any more food and goes into starvation mode. At that point it basically stops using our excess fat.

Tests have shown that there are additional health benefits to intermittent fasting. These include increasing insulin sensitivity, reducing oxidative stress, and increase the capacity for resisting cellular stress. All of these will retard aging of the cells as well as preventing diseases associated with cell damage. So is an intermittent fasting plan right for everyone? Actually, all of the factors that go into healthy weight reduction make it nearly impossible to find one magic bullet that will be right for everyone. First, it is safe to say that pregnant women should never fast. A baby needs all the nutrients they can get, and some studies have actually suggested that fasting can alter the baby's heartbeat and breathing patterns, along with increasing gestational diabetes. Those that suffer from hypoglycemia, a condition of abnormally lower level of blood sugar, should not go through periods of fasting. Your goal if you have this condition would be to normalize your blood sugar levels first, then if you decide to fast opt for a less rigid version of fasting. Those with diabetes also will not be helped with intermittent fasting.

You must realize that if you are going too fast, you must pay even more attention to your nutrition levels when you do eat. By continuing with a toxic-rich diet of highly processed foods, then proceed to not eat for 15 or 16 hours, you could be doing your body more harm than good in the long run. Putting together a healthy diet plan to make sure you are getting the proper nutrition in the shorter time period you are eating in will be vital. Whenever you are going to make dramatic changes in your diet, even if they are healthy changes that will eventually greatly benefit your health, it may take a little while for your system to adjust to the change. But listen to what your body is telling you, and if you are going a little too quickly, don't fight it. Just go a bit slower with the changes, and if it is good for your system will eventually adapt. Tapping into fat storage is one of the secrets to weight loss. It not only requires good diet and exercise, but there is evidence that what you eat and timing when you eat is important.

Why You Should Try Intermittent Fasting

Intermittent fasting is a controversial weight loss technique because it involves not eating food for an extended period of time. Many people have the notion that not eating will slow down your metabolism and send your body into starvation mode, but it turns out this is not true at all. In fact, the human body was designed to go long periods of time without eating, so intermittent fasting is actually a natural practice. Perhaps that is why it is so

effective. If you would like to lose weight but don't want to give up certain foods or don't want to partake in vigorous exercise, intermittent fasting is probably your best option. Fasting will help you lose weight quickly, even if you don't eat extremely healthy or exercise, although that would greatly enhance your results. This technique doesn't even require you to lower the amount of calories you consume. It simply takes a little bit of discipline in the beginning.

If you don't like the idea of fasting, perhaps the benefits will convince you to give it a try anyway. Intermittent fasting has many benefits that will greatly increase the quality of your life. Some of the benefits include:

- Rapid fat loss

- Lowered blood pressure and cholesterol

- Increase in energy, especially in the mornings

- Enhanced memory and cognitive ability

These are just a few of the many benefits that fasting can offer you. If you simply want to be a healthier and/or happier person, it would be of your best interest to begin an intermittent fasting routine. So, how can you begin?

There are a few ways one can begin fasting. One method, the one I prefer, is daily fasting. This involves eating your food for the day within a time period of 6 to 8 hours. This would mean you fast for 16 to 18 hours every day. The easiest way to do this is to skip breakfast in the mornings. You will benefit greatly from this. Even greater benefits will be experienced when you can lengthen the time spent fasting. For example, fast for 20 hours and eat for 4. Figure out what works best for you. Another method that also works well is weekly fasting. This would involve a period of fasting that lasts between 24 and 36 hours. So, for example, you would eat as you normally do for 6 days of the week, then one day you would not eat any food at all. Drink plenty of water during the time when you are not eating. Weekly fasting is also effective, but not as effective as daily fasting I have found. I encourage you to learn more and begin to incorporate one of these strategies into your life.

Intermittent Fasting - How to Do It Healthily and Safely

Intermittent fasting can improve health, reduce the risk of serious illness, and promote longevity. Perhaps you're intrigued and would like to give it a go but aren't sure how to start. Or maybe you have tried it once or twice and found it too challenging. This book will give you strategies and guidelines to practice intermittent fasting safely and successfully. Please read the contraindications at the end of this article before doing a fast. There are three main ways to do intermittent fasting - a) only eat from 6pm to bedtime every day, b) a 24-hour fast on alternate days, or c) one or two 36-hour fasts each week. It's worth experimenting with all 3 strategies to see which works best for you in terms of your lifestyle and effect on your health and wellbeing. The guidelines I've given you below are mainly for the 36hr fast, but most are helpful for the 24hr fast as well.

Pick a day that isn't too hectic or demanding because you may experience some detox reactions. Make sure you have the option to relax if you need to. You will get more out of the experience if you make time to turn inward, still the mind, meditate, contemplate, and listen to your inner guidance. Enlist Support from people close to

<table>
<tr><td>

About fat loss supplements

They don't work. Yep, fat loss supplements are a huge waste of money. They don't speed up your metabolism or anything. In fact most of them just suppress your appetite so you eat less. Appetite suppression is something you can control with sheer will power so why pay money for it?

</td></tr>
</table>

you before you start. It's great to fast with your partner so you can both motivate each other and share experiences. Eat lightly the evening before by choosing a large salad or steamed vegetables with some lean protein. There is no point gorging the night before because it will make you feel even hungrier whilst you fast. It's best to avoid alcohol as well. Keep hydrated during the fast as your body has an essential need for fluid. Water, herbal teas, and vegetable juices are good choices. Have at least 2 litres of fluid during the day. Avoid coffee, tea, fizzy drinks, fruit juice, and alcohol. Have 1 or 2 glasses of vegetable juice as it will provide important electrolytes as well as having a health-boosting alkalizing effect. Try juicing celery, cucumber, chicory, fennel, and watercress. Avoid carrots and beets as they are quite high in sugar. Don't fight feeling hungry because you most probably will. Just be with the sensation without judgment, rather than resisting it (but read guideline 10 below).

Engage in light exercise such as walking, stretching, and gentle yoga. This is not the day to do an intense gym workout or anything too vigorous. Add some breathing exercises such as yogic pranayama. A few minutes of practice offer amazing benefits from detoxification to boosting energy. Expect some detox symptoms such as headaches, feeling groggy, or short periods of feeling jittery. These are made worse if you usually have lots of caffeine and sugar in your diet. Avoid taking over-the-counter medication to reduce these side effects. Instead rest, go for a walk, and practice breathing exercises. Listen to your body wisdom and if you feel unwell or it gets too much then have some food. Your body knows best. Break the fast gently the following morning. Have water or herb tea and a piece of fruit when you get up then 30min later have your usual breakfast. Eat as usual for the rest of the day (you probably won't feel the need to overeat). Enjoy the changes in how you feel during and after the fast. Notice changes in your energy, emotions, and mental state. You may notice food is far more enjoyable on the day after the fast because your senses are heightened. Recognise that it can take a few attempts to get used to this practice. After a few weeks your body will get used to it and the benefits you feel will increase as the discomfort simultaneously decreases.

The essential for a successful intermittent fasting program

- Dedication
- Determination
- Your body
- A good exercise program

What you don't need

- You will not need to buy specific foods, eat what you want to but remember moderation is the key factor.

- You will not need a personal trainer if you are well-versed in training. If you are not you may seek out a trainer or consult the inter net for information.

- You don't need any shady fat burning supplements.

The Wonderful Benefits of Intermittent Fasting

The pattern of eating called "Intermittent Fasting" usually means one fasts for a period of time and eats for a period of time. Many choose a 24 hour cycle of fasting, then eat healthy the next day, and continue this process as a lifestyle change. Research has been done on animals to find the benefits of this type of fasting, and you will be happy to know it really can be beneficial to your health!Intermittent fasting can add 40%-56%

more years to your life! That in itself is reason enough to do it.

However other benefits include body weight reduction and fat oxidation. When you fast your body is forced to scavenge for fuel thus removing aged and damaged cells in the process. This sort of cleanses the body of undesirable and unwanted things and helps the weight loss and benefits of the good food choices be increased and more beneficial to your body. Rats have been shown to have long-term and improved survival after heart failure after being on a IF eating plan, too. Researchers are also saying that it might help age related deficits in cognitive function, too, so that tells me that it might help ward off

Alzheimer's Disease and other types of Dementia!

Your risk of heart disease and other heart ailments may also be decreased when you start a healthy intermittent fasting regimen. Your risk for other chronic illnesses and diseases will also most likely be reduced. A healthier you can begin with intermittent fasting and healthy food choices. Keep carbs to 50-100 grams per day. Many women eat between 1200-1500 calories per day, and when limiting their carbs, they are still losing weight. Men can handle up to 2000 calories per day. Of course less is best, and you need to determine caloric intake based on your activity such as working hard and exercising.

Drink lots of fluids, especially water and exercise in the evenings if possible. This will help with those late night cravings. Once you start eating and drinking healthier, your body won't crave as much (if any) junk food, so making healthy food choices will simply get easier and easier as you progress in the intermittent fasting routine. Alternate Day Fasting or ADF means alternating days of eating and not eating any food, but there is also an intermittent fasting called Modified Fasting where you consume about 20% of your normal calories one day and then eat normally (but healthy) the next day. This is often more attainable for people because they feel less deprived when they are able to at least eat something daily, and it still has most of the benefits of the ADF regimen. Whatever you choose to do, make sure you tell your health care professional of your plans so he or she is aware and can work with you to reach your goals. If you want to lose weight, lose fat and feel better, then intermittent fasting might be the answer for you!

One of the hormones in your body is called IGF-1 (insulin-like growth factor 1); it helps your cells grow and is particularly important in growing children. As you reach adulthood, however, it decreases significantly. This is important, since as you grow older it appears to have adverse effects: it accelerates aging and can even lead to cancer. So it's not something you want high levels of when you're older. And studies have shown that intermittent fasting decreases it.

Also, in your brain is a protein referred to as BDNF (brain-derived neurotrophic factor). It is important because it has been shown to help stem cells turn into new neurons. This takes place in a section of the brain called the hippocampus, which is critical in relation to memory and learning, BDNF has many effects: it appears to protect against dementia and Alzheimer's disease, and it also acts as an anti-depressant, suppressing anxiety. Intermittent fasting also helps increase autophagy, which is a system in the cells that gets rid of damaged molecules that could lead to serious neurological diseases.

Diabetes

Diabetes comes in two forms: diabetes I and diabetes II. We will be mainly concerned with diabetes II. As we saw earlier, all cells use glucose as fuel. But it can't get into the cells without insulin. Insulin is produced in the pancreas according to the amount of glucose in the blood; it's role is to allow the glucose to enter the cell. Most of the cells in your body have what are called insulin receptors that bind to insulin that is circulating in your blood. When a cell has insulin attached to its surface it allows glucose in, so it obviously plays an important role in your body. But too much can be detrimental. Insulin increases your hunger, promotes the storage of fat cells, and it has been linked to diabetes and heart problems. One of the major problems associated with insulin is what is called insulin resistance. In this case the pancreas produces insulin, but insulin receptors on the cells no longer work properly, and don't allow glucose to enter as they should. With no place to go, the glucose continues to circulate in the blood, and the cells soon begin to starve. The body realizes that something is wrong and the pancreas produces more insulin in an attempt to get sucrose into the cells, but this causes the pancreas to overwork, and it eventually begins to wear out. The result is diabetes II.

Studies have shown that intermittent fasting improves your insulin sensitivity. This in turn allows your body to do a better job of controlling your blood glucose levels after meals, and therefore helps rest your pancreas. Both of these are important in relation to the prevention of diabetes II.

Rules for Fasting

- It is best to use a 5 - 2 approach, with regular meals 5 days a week, and two days of restricted food (500 calories for women, 600 for men).

- Stay hydrated. Drink Plenty of water; it helps flush out toxins.

- When not on fasting days (and even when fasting), keep your nutrition maximized. In particular, eat sufficient vegetables, fruits and whole grains.

- Remember that 12 hours of fasting is needed for the effect. From 12 to 18 hours is best. It plateau's beyond 18.

- You can exercise during fasting periods, but don't overdo it.

- Be careful of fasting if you are diabetic.

Chapter Two

The Truth About Fasting

The following information can be applied to any diet. Before you start any diet it is important that you familiarize yourself with the basics of a diet.

The Truth About Fasting

The benefits of fasting have been big news lately. But how effective is it? Most people are interested in it as a weight loss tool, and indeed you can lose weight using it, but in reality it has many benefits beyond weight loss, and some of them are quite miraculous. It has been known for many years that it extends the life of mice, worms and flies rather dramatically, and even appears to extend the life of monkeys. Does it extend the life of humans? Many people are convinced that it does, but the truth is that we're still not sure, although it looks hopeful. There's no doubt, however, that it has health benefits in relation to heart disease, cancer, dementia, and even your mood and well-being. It can't be called a cure, but it does set the stage for healing by allowing vital parts of your body to rest and recuperate. There's no doubt that excess eating puts a burden on your body, and that it needs an occasional rest. Indeed, studies have shown that if it doesn't rest, it forgoes much of the repair and regeneration needed for optimal health.

Glucose, Glycogen and Fat

Your body needs energy to run properly, and it gets this energy from the food you eat. Food is turned a form of sugar called glucose. Your cells (and particularly the ones in your brain) need a constant supply of glucose, and if it gets low you begin to feel fatigued and weak.

Glucose circulates in your blood after you eat, and it is used up fairly rapidly as you go about your everyday tasks. If not replenished, it is, in fact, depleted in a few hours. This creates a problem: how do you maintain a good supply? Glucose itself can't be stored, but it can be turned into a form called glycogen that can be stored in your muscles and liver. From here it can be drawn out and used as needed. It is usually good for about 10 to 12 hours. What happens when it is depleted? The body then turns to the fat cells that are stored throughout your body. They can be broken down and converted to what is called ketones. This is, of course, what dieters look for, namely, the loss of fat cells. But you have to be careful if you remain in this stage for too long. The body soon begins to break down protein; it can also be converted to glucose through a rather complicated process. And this causes the loss of muscle - something you don't want. Indeed, in most diets, a fair amount of the weight loss comes from muscle loss along with depletion of water (leaving you dehydrated). So don't be deceived.

Weight Loss Through Fasting

As it was mentioned earlier, you can lose weight by fasting, but most doctors and dieticians do not recommend long fasting periods because they can have an adverse effect on your overall health. In addition, it is difficult for most people to fast for long periods of time. A better alternative is what is called intermittent fasting in which you fast on certain days of the week, and eat normally on the others. One form of this is alternate-day fasting. In this case you fast (or restrict your calories) on one day and eat normally the next. This works well for some people but Dr. Michael Mosley of BBC has put forward what he calls the 5-2 fasting diet. In this diet you restrict your calories only two days a week. He suggests 500 calories for women on these days and 600 for men. This is much easier for most people to do, and it appears to give the same results as more extended fasts. But weight loss is not the most important benefit of such a diet, so let's look at the other benefits.

How does weight loss occur?

Weight loss is a process of being in a caloric deficit. A caloric deficit is when you use more calories than you are consuming. Weight loss cannot occur without a caloric deficit. Go back and read the last sentence until you have fully grasped the concept of weight loss.

What if I want to gain weight?

Since weight loss occurs when we are not consuming enough calories to meet our daily use, then weight gain is the opposite. Weight gain occurs when we exceed our daily caloric needs thus the extra calories are stored as fat. If you induce a stimulus such as weight training than the extra calories will be used to repair and improve the damaged muscles thus enlarging your muscles and ultimately results in you gaining muscle weight.

Preserving Muscle

You always hear people saying "I want to lose weight" or "I need to lose some weight" but they never specify what type of weight. Muscle contributes to your total bodyweight too, so does water, and your organs and so on. You could lose

Why IF Works

As you know by now losing weight is all about being in a negative calorie deficit. In a typical IF program you will fast for the majority of the day. Then you may have one meal at the end of the day.

So even if you attempt to overeat during that one meal you will be full way before you reach your daily caloric intake. Thus you will be in a constant negative deficit.

10lbs of muscle, but would you be satisfied?

The correct phrase is "I want to lose fat".

Typically fat (adipose tissue) is what most people are referring to when they want to lose weight. However what inevitable happens during a diet is muscle loss.

Here's why.

Muscles are calorically expensive. Think of it as a bank. Say each pound of lean muscle requires 25 calories to uphold. So if 100lbs of your total bodyweight is pure muscle than you need to eat 2,500 calories a day just to maintain your muscle mass. Say now you want to go on a diet so you reduce your calories down 2,300. Now a problem arises. You don't have enough calories to maintain your muscle mass. Still using the bank analogy, you are now presented with two choices you can sell off your muscle (break down muscle tissue to pay for the other muscles and reduce total spending) or you can take out a loan (break down fatty tissue for extra calories).

Ideally you want the latter because that's what fat is for right? Fat is to be used as energy when we are in a deficit.

So then how does muscle loss occur? Muscle loss occurs when we exceed our loan limit. Say our deficit is now 1500 calories and we still need 2500 calories each day. We find ourselves down 1000 calories however we can only take out a max loan of 500 calories from our fat reserves. This limit occurs because there is a limit to which fat can be broken down. Thus we are force to breakdown some of our muscle to pay for the rest. So in conclusion to minimize muscle losses always reduce your daily calorie needs by small increments (200 or 100 calories) so that you don't exceed

Your Body Is Amazing At Survival

Back during the ice age era our ancestors would go days without eating. They lived their life not knowing when their next meal would be or what it will come from.

So our body is well-adapted for survival. This is why our body stores fat, to have an extra storage of calories when we are starving. Fat is our insurance. Another reason why our body prefers breakdown our muscle is that it sees that it can reduce daily spending by getting rid of the calorie expensive things such as muscle.

However our ancestor didn't have to worry about losing muscle because their lifestyle was more active. They had to run, jump, climb trees, scale mountains, throw spears, carry the old and wounded, and so on. So their body's top priority was to keep their muscle or else they wouldn't survive in such a world.

Fast forward to today and a majority of us lead sedentary lifestyles. Our body says "oh it's okay for us to get rid of these muscles, it's not like we use it for anything". That's where weight training comes in. Weight training gives our body a reason to keep our hard-earned muscles.

Remember our body adapts to make life easier

your loan limit. Utilize a strength training program to ensure that your body realizes that your muscles are needed.

Are all calories equal?

Yes are calories are equal. There is no such thing as good food and bad food just food that are more calorie dense (higher in calories) and food that are lower in calories. If you still have doubts about a calorie being a calorie, go read <u>about the professor who lost 27 pounds while eating only Twinkies.</u>

All calories are equal, but are all foods equal?

I said earlier that there aren't such things as good foods or bad foods well that was a lie.

There are foods that are filled to the brim with man-made chemicals such as high fructose corn syrup. These chemicals are potentially harmful and thus should be avoided or kept to a minimum. As a general rule the closer the food is to its natural form, the better. I am not saying that you can't enjoy your favorite foods but simply stating that the majority of your diet should consist of natural foods. The benefits of a healthy diet are endless but here are a few

- Higher energy levels

- Better mood

- Less risk of diseases

- Stronger immune system

- Healthier skin

- Stronger bones

- Longer life

Macronutrients and Caloric Maintenance

I won't delve too much into this topic as there is a wealth of information on the internet and it would be outside the scope of this manual. So consider this a brief introduction to macronutrients.

Macronutrients are protein, carbohydrates, and lipids (fats).

Protein: If you are a serious weight lifter or an athlete then you should be aware of the importance of protein. Proteins are the building block of muscle and any aid in recovery after a training session. Of the three (carbs, fats, and protein) protein is the most important. Protein can be found in meats, dairy, nuts, and legumes (beans). The general rule for any athlete is 1 gram of protein per pound of bodyweight. For example if you weigh 150lbs than you should strive to eat 150 grams of protein per day. Each gram of protein is equivalent to approximately 4 calories.

Carbohydrates: Carbohydrates are your body's main source of energy. The majority of your daily calories will come in the form of carbohydrates. Carbohydrates come in two major forms, sugars and starches. Sugars are easily digested and thus enter the blood stream immediately. Starches take a while to digest and are often stored in the muscles as glycogen. Each gram of carbohydrate is equivalent to approximately 4 calories.

Examples of carbohydrates are bread, pasta, grain, sugar, potatoes, and rice.

Fats: The media has completely destroyed the reputation of fats and thus when we hear the word we often associate it with synonyms such as "bad". However fats are not all bad and some fat is necessary for optimal health. There are three types of fats, saturated, unsaturated and trans. Generally trans-fat are bad and increase your risk of heart disease. Saturated fats are not necessary bad but should be limited to a small percent of your diet. Foods with saturated fats are meat, butter, lard, cream, etc.

Unsaturated fats have been proven to decrease your risk of developing heart disease. You can include unsaturated fats into your diet by consuming foods such as avocados, nuts and any food cooked with olive oil.

Caloric Maintenance: caloric maintenance is simply the number of calories your body needs in day to maintain homeostasis, which is to have no weight gain or weight loss but to stay at equilibrium. Caloric maintenance varies with each individual. It may be higher if you are younger, more active, and have more muscle mass. Your caloric maintenance will be achieved through a combination of protein, carbohydrates and fats. Generally for new trainees I recommend a standard 40/40/20 ratio which means 40% protein,

40% carbohydrates and 20% fats. For example I generally eat around 3000 calories a day to maintain my bodyweight. So 40% of 3000 is 1200 calories. 1200 divided by 4 is 300 grams of protein. If I followed a 40/40/20 ratio then my diet would be the following.

3000 calories (40/40/20)	Protein 40%	Carbohydrates 40%	Fats 20%
calories	1200	1200	600
grams	300g	300g	67g

It should be noted that consuming 300grams of protein in one day is next to impossible as that would mean you would have to chug down copious amounts of protein shakes. Thus a more realistic macronutrient ratio would be a 20/60/20 ratio. See below for an example.

3000 calories (20/60/20)	Protein 20%	Carbohydrates 60%	Fats 20%
calories	600	1800	600
grams	150g	450g	67g

To determine your caloric maintenance a good starting point would be to use a daily calorie calculator. You can find many calorie calculators online such as the one at Freedieting.com. My suggestion is to use the calculator to obtain an estimate. Then test the estimate for two weeks if you happen to gain weight subtract a little, such as 200 calories from the estimate and retest for another two weeks. If you lose weight than try adding 200 calories to the estimate and keep testing until you find your caloric maintenance. I know this task is meticulous and often frustrating when you have to carry a calorie log everywhere you go. Even then there will be times when you will not be able to know how much calories is in the meal you consumed.

However the good news is that with enough experience you will eventually be able to accurately guess how much calorie certain foods consume. For example I am now able to eye-ball foods and obtain a good estimate of how much calorie was in the meal I ate.

Starvation vs. Hunger

A common mistake to make during a diet is to confuse hunger with starvation. People will often feel their stomach growling and assume that if they don't eat soon they will vaporize into thin air. Well I was kidding about the vaporizing, but people will often pre-maturely end their fast because their stomach was rumbling. The premise is that once your body enters starvation mode your metabolism rate drops thus you will burn less calories and your diet will be in vain. However that is not the case. Studies on fasting and metabolism has shown that the earliest sign of a decrease in metabolism occurs after 60 hours and none of the IF programs will have you fasting more than 24 hours so you won't have to worry about a reduced metabolism. So what do I do about the hunger pangs? From personal experience I found that if you just ignore them and continue about your day the hunger will go away immediately. However do not mistake hunger with physical pain. If your stomach is in physical pain and actually hurts then you are doing something wrong. Please consult a physician. The good news is that if you follow the IF methods that I have listed in chapter 2 you will never have physical stomach pain.

An interesting phenomenon that I learn about hunger is that you are able to control hunger. Before I started using intermittent fasting I use to eat 6 meals a day. You know the whole "if you eat more you will increase your metabolism nonsense" which has been proven wrong in case you were wondering. During my six meals a day diet I normally ate at 8:00am. 11:00am, 2:00pm, 5:00pm, 8:00pm and 11:00pm. So during the first week of intermittent fasting I would become hungry around the same times because my body was so used to eating at those times. However I ignored my hunger and by my third week of IF my tolerance for hunger was slowly dissipating and I could go longer without eating. Not only that but I would only feel hungry during the feeding window of my intermittent fasting program. So what's the moral of the story? You are in the master of your hunger.

Chapter Three

Intermittent Fasting Results: What You Can Expect

Intermittent fasting is a feeding pattern which alternates between periods of fasting and controlled eating. It is a simple dietary method divided into many types. One of the intermittent fasting methods is alternate day fasting, whereby a person takes a normal diet on particular days of the week and fasts on some. During the fasting days, one does not fully abstain from food but rather reduces calorie intake to 1/4 of the normal diet. The other fasting type is whereby eating is restricted to a certain time window within a day. This means restricting eating between an 8 hour window eating period, which means a person eats once in every eight hours. Some people however reduce the span to either six, four or even two hours according to their convenience. The longest time that a person can stay without food on intermittent fasting is 36 hours. If practiced accordingly, it can result in a number of positive health effects. For instance, intermittent fasting promotes general good health. It significantly reduces cravings for snack foods and sugars. The practice normalizes insulin as well as leptin sensitivity. Insulin resistance contributes to many chronic diseases such as diabetes, cancer and heart infections. Intermittent fasting will therefore protect the body from such infections.

Intermittent fasting results in improved brain health. Fasting helps the body to convert stored glycogen into glucose to release energy. If the fasting proceeds for some time, continued breakdown of body fats induces the liver to secrete ketone bodies. These small molecules are by-products of fatty acids synthesis, and the brain can use them as fuel. Research also indicates that exercise and fasting results in genes and other growth factors which are essential in recycling and rejuvenating the brain.

This type of fasting also boosts body fitness and loss of weight. Combined fasting and exercise increases effects of catalysts and cellular factors so that breakdown of glycogen and fats is maximized. Exercising while hungry therefore forces the body to burn stored fats for significant weight loss. The program is also known to prevent cognitive decline. Research was conducted in 2006 on mice, in which water maze tests were used to assess cognitive functions of mice on normal diet and those on intermittent fasting. It was discovered that mice put on intermittent fasting experienced slower cognitive declines, which too applies to human beings.

Intermittent fasting will also boost muscle building especially in men. This is because after eating, the energy gained will be used to sustain a workout session. But if training is done while fasting, the body utilizes stored body fats to sustain the exercises. Eating after the session ensures that the energy gained is utilized in replenishing the body in the best way. This assists the muscles to quickly recover and build up.

Weekly Diet Plan: Why You Should Add Intermittent Fasting

It seems as though everyone is on a diet and rightfully so, since the majority of people are obese. How did it come to this? Can anything be done to snap the nation back into shape and jump start a weekly diet plan? Chances are no one has heard of intermittent fasting as a way to burn fat but has heard of fasting for religious purposes. Many religions include obligatory fasting as a way to purify the body in a spiritual sense such as the Islamic religion and its month of Ramadan. But, can fasting be used as a way to cleanse the body and lose weight simultaneously? It certainly can and recently people have been using this method to trim unwanted inches on their tummies and waistlines.

Benefits of Fasting

Recent studies on fasting show the benefits to be:

- Reduction in glucose levels
- Increase in growth hormone
- Fat burning

- Glucagon increase (helps in burning fat)

- Reduction in inflammation

- Detoxification

Many people are opposed to fasting as they believe they must constantly eat to maintain their metabolism. This is simply not true. In clinical studies, it was determined the body's metabolism is directly related to the amount of lean body mass or muscle on the individual. Those with less muscle will have a slower metabolism as opposed to those who are more muscular. It doesn't have anything to do with frequency or volume of meals as food companies would want the general public to believe.

Weekly Diet Plan Plus : The bonuses to following your weekly diet plan and adding intermittent fasting into it are numerous. First, you'll save on food bills. Since you're

Here are some guidelines to follow when fasting:

- Fast on non-consecutive days - so if you intermittent fast on Monday then don't attempt to fast again until Wednesday
- Don't stuff yourself after fasting (you'll be tempted to over eat but don't)
- Don't eat excessively sugary foods when coming off the fast
- Drink plenty of water while fasting (especially if you begin to feel hungry, drinking extra water will help)
- Coffee helps to curb appetite, so have a cup of "joe" on the morning of your fast, but don't add sugar as it will break the fast. Bonus: Use

eating less, there will be fewer trips to the grocery store or restaurant. Second, you won't have to think about or prepare what you're going to eat that day. Our lives are constantly consumed with asking ourselves, **"What am I going to eat**?" Wouldn't it be nice to not have to think about it? In addition, by adding IF to your diet plan, you'll finally be able to control the urge to eat which is half the battle in trying to lose pounds and inches. IF should be an integral part of your weekly diet plan if it isn't already. There's no better method than IF to cut calories easily and gain immense health benefits.

Keys to Understanding Intermittent Fasting

With intermittent fasting becoming more and more popular as a weight-loss and health management diet, it is important to understand how to set it up; here are keys to make sure that you can get involved in an intermittent fasting lifestyle as soon as possible.

- Intermittent fasting doesn't need to be a short term approach to dieting and is in fact much more successful as a genuine lifestyle choice. The first decision to make therefore is how to adapt a fast to YOUR life. Remember that the fast can be anywhere from 16 hours to several days in length depending on exactly what you are trying to accomplish. The two approaches that are perhaps easiest to set up are an alternating day (24 hour) fast/eat cycle, or a 16/8 cycle.

- When do I workout? This question is key. Diet is with doubt the most important factor in weight-loss and good health, but to really get the best out of an intermittent fast, the re-feed should coincide with your workout. Personally, I have had good success with a fast from 8Pm until the next day at lunch and an early afternoon training session. All the food that I am taking in around my workout is being used for fuel and to repair muscle rather than being stocked as body-fat.

- What do I want to accomplish with intermittent fasting? Is your aim fat-loss, muscle gain, improved health or a combination of all three? Depending on your answer to these questions, you can start to identify exactly how long your fast should be and what quantity of food your should be eating during the eating "window".

How to Setup an Intermittent Fasting Diet

Here is the extremely basic summary of how it works:

- On training days, eat 9 hours of the day and fast the remaining 15.
- On off or cardio days, eat 6 hours of the day and fast the remaining 18.
- Weight training 3 days per week
- Cardio 2-4 times per week
- Eat maintenance + 500 calories on weight training days
- Eat 50% of maintenance on other days
- Majority of carbohydrate intake is on weight training days.

Again, this plan is specific to fat loss. Plans for mass gain (bulking) and maintenance will be coming soon. Now for the detailed explanation of:

How to set up an Intermittent Fasting Diet for Fat Loss

Establishing Eating / Fasting Times

The time of day in which you eat depends on if you are lifting weights that day, or not. On lifting days, your eating window is 9 hours and on off or cardio days, its 6 hours. You will need to be able to weight train and do cardio at the same time of day, as this will throw off the schedule.

Eating schedule for weight training days

The fast is broken by a pre-workout shake, 15-30 minutes before you being your workout and lasts for 9 hours. For example, since I workout at 1pm, my eating window begins at 12:30 pm and lasts until 9:30 pm. This can be inconvenient if you workout at say, 8pm, so I feel weightlifting at lunchtime or in the morning works best. The fast is broken an hour after cardio is complete and lasts for 6 hours. In my case, I do cardio at 1pm, so my fast is broken at 3pm. It remains 3pm on off days.

Chapter Four

Intermittent Fasting Programs

How Can I Lose A Stone In A Month - Rapid Weight Loss With Intermittent Fasting

- **How much food do you need?**

Or more specifically, how much protein should you be aiming for at each meal? Well, we can give two answers to that question, the answer that's best is the one that makes you feel most reassured. The quick answer is 'lots'. The more specific answer is worked out as follows; start with a level of about 1g/lb of bodyweight and divide over your two or three meals, and then adjust based on lean tissue and strength drops and hunger/satiety levels. So if you find your strength dropping, and your muscle leaving your body, you need to add more protein in, and if you find yourself getting hungry between meals or not satisfied at a meal, add more protein!

- **What Foods Can I Eat?**

I've put together a list of foods that will work whilst eating for massive fat loss. You can download it from my website, via the link at the bottom. One thing that I consistently find is the total lack of hunger and feelings of deprivation when on this type of diet, and this shouldn't be surprising given the huge range of foods on offer here. One thing you'll notice is the total lack of liquid foods/meal replacement powders/protein drinks. This is deliberate; they don't provide satiety and satisfaction, and they don't offer much opportunity for long term diet adherence. As Martin Berkhan says, 'don't drink your calories'.

- **Why High Protein, Low Fat, Low Carb?**

A couple of reasons; 1, you want to keep calories as low as possible, as easily as possible. 2, protein plus lots of bulky yet low carb density foods provides the easiest way to feel full, satisfied and happy when cutting calories.

- Doing only high intensity weights and very low intensity cardio

Each of the three components in this weight loss plan are equally important, so you'd better find a way of including this part! Just ask yourself if it's worth jeopardising the whole plan for the sake of missing some simple exercises?

Why start with a statement like that?

Because it's too easy for many people to drop back into old ways of 'exercising for weight loss'.

What you NEED to be doing is heavy weights, with low reps and using as big movements as possible. Remember, big weights are totally specific to each individual, and the actual number/weight is irrelevant, what's important is that you lift to YOUR capacity and you learn how to fully lift at your capacity. For those of you that have hardly lifted weights before that means learning what a max effort lift feels like, AND expecting that max to go up quickly as you learn how to get more and more out of yourself.

The great thing about this program is that it really is simple. Take the following exercises and rotate them:

- *Squat*

- *Dumbell press, bench press or bodyweight dips*

- *Dumbell or barbell shoulder press*

- *Lat pulldown, pullup, seated row or bent over barbell/dumbell row*

- *Deadlift.*

Your rotation is simple: Do 3 weeks of 5set sof 4-6 reps (5x5 style routine) and then 3 weeks of 3 sets of 9-12 reps (3x10 style routine). Each time you hit the upper rep range you increase the weight. Only after 10-14 weeks do you need to rest (but if you've already been exercising consistently for more than 12 weeks, you need to take a week of total rest right now - unless you're goal is within 12 weeks from the start of your program, in which case, you get your rest at the end of that!)

The 24 Hour Fast (24 hour fast once a week)

Popularized by Brad Pilon author of Eat Stop Eat, the 24 hour fast is a fast that lasts an entire day. You will only fast on one day of the week and on the other 6 days you will eat normally. The 24 hour fast views fat loss in a weekly basis. For example if you normally eat 2000 calories per day that is a total of 14,000 calories a week. Now if you subtract one day then you are down to 12,000 calories.

Who is this approach for?

The 24 hour fast works great for beginners and casual dieters. It is the easiest of all the programs because there is only one rule to follow. People who are new to IF should start with the 24 fast and work their way to the other IF programs if desired.

Rules

1. Don't eat for 24 hours

Instructions

1. Pick a day you would like to fast on

2. Set the beginning time for your fast for example if you decide that your last meal should be at 8:00pm on Wednesday than you will fast until 8:00pm on Thursday

3. Be productive on your fast day and get your work done.

What not to do

- Don't compensate by eating more on the other 6 days. If you do find yourself eating more, know that you have some space for cushion. For example if you ate an extra 400 calories on Friday know that you are still in a deficit of 1600 (2000-400) so do not worry.

- Don't think about food during your fast. Keep your mind occupied

What Makes Intermittent Fasting Different?

Intermittent fasting weight loss is one of the most effective ways to shed off your extra pounds. The ideas on intermittent fasting weight loss challenge most of the previously held beliefs on losing. Those who are seeking new ways to lose weight effectively have quickly embraced its ideas.

What is Intermittent Fasting Weight Loss?

Let start by clarifying that intermittent fasting is not a diet. You are probably tired of trying anything with the word 'diet' on it when it comes to weight loss. Intermittent fasting is a way of eating that involves a structured program on the times when you eat and when you do not eat. You structure your program according to your fancy. If you can handle it, fast for a whole day!

What Makes it Different?

If you have tried to lose weight, you probably have tried diets such as Atkins diet based on the frequent feeding theory. Simply, proponents of such diets told you to eat often during the day. The idea was that the more you eat, the faster your metabolism. The faster your metabolism, the more fat you will lose. Of course, you do know that the more you ate, the more you wanted to eat and the more your weight remained. When you are on an intermittent program, you will have to cut down your meal frequency. Sometimes, you have to do without breakfast.

Tell Me More

You probably sleep for around 6 to 8 hours. During this time, your body is in fasting mode. When your body is in fasting mode, it usually produces more insulin. More insulin in your body causes your body to have increased insulin sensitivity. When your body has increased insulin sensitivity, you lose more fat. The brilliance of intermittent fasting weight loss program is that you skip breakfast to extend the period of your body's insulin sensitivity. This means that your body is going to be on fat loss mode for a longer period. You will lose more weight.

A longer fasting mode also has a good effect on the Growth hormone levels in your body. By skipping breakfast or eating during a specific period, your body produces Growth hormone. Growth hormone is what you want your body producing when you are trying to lose weight. This is simply because Growth hormone promotes weight loss in your body. When you are on an intermittent fasting weight loss program, your Growth hormone levels are usually at their peak. You will be losing more weight during this period. High Growth hormone levels in your body also have several other health benefits. This program is simply amazing!

Intermittent fasting weight loss program is radically different from most weight loss programs being promoted in the market. However, its ideas are scientifically sound when it comes to losing weight. You should give this program a go if you are serious about weight loss.

Commonly Asked Questions About Intermittent Fasting and Supplements

- **What is the most important supplement that I should be taking?**

At bare minimum, everyone should be taking a multivitamin of some sort because of nutrient deficient soil. I prefer organic, whole food vitamin sources such as powdered greens.

- **What supplements should I be taking?**

A multivitamin, an omega 3 source, a probiotic, and Vitamin D. As I said before, I prefer whole food sources over artificial multivitamins. So I would use a greens source as my multivitamin. I use a high quality fish oil or krill oil for my omega 3 source. An alternative for vegans would be flaxseed oil or hemp oil. As for probiotics, the best source is naturally fermented foods such as miso soup, kimchi, natto, kefir, and sauerkraut. As for supplementation, get one that has more than 10 billion active probiotic strains per serving. Vitamin D supplementation is very important for people who don't get one hour of sunlight exposure per day. For instance, if you live in the northeast US, you will definitely need it. People with darker complexions will need more sun exposure than light skinned folks because UV-B rays do not penetrate the skin as far. Therefore, less sunlight is converted to Vitamin D. The latest studies are saying that almost everyone is deficient in Vitamin D.

- **What is the best type of protein powder to buy?**

It depends on what you are using it for. Whey is the best all-purpose protein. It absorbs fast, is cheap, and is best taken after a workout. Casein protein is best taken before bed because it is slowly absorbed. I would stick to a protein powder that is made from grass-fed cow's milk for higher quality.

- **When should I take my protein supplement: before or after a workout?**

If you can afford it, both. The influx of branch chained amino acids taken before will give you a better performance throughout your workout. If you are trying to save money, the optimal time to take a protein supplement is within 30 minutes of completing your workout for recovery.

- **I have tried all diets and they have failed. What's the easiest way to see results without dieting?**

Intermittent fasting may work for you. Research shows that the 18th hour is the "golden hour". This is when you see the most results for the least amount of time. There are different theories on intermittent fasting. Some say the fast starts after your last meal and others say that it starts 2 or 3 hours after your last meal due to digestion. You do not want to fast over 24 hours straight. This is where negative effects on metabolism are seen and honestly anything over 24 hours is miserable and uncomfortable.

Reasons Why You Should Consider Intermittent Fasting - Apart From Weight Loss

So you want to lose weight and you have chosen to lose weight by intermittent fasting. For those of you who don't know, intermittent fasting is simply a system that alternates between periods of eating and not eating (usually you get to consume water and sometimes low-calorie drinks such as black coffee).

What this means is that for a set time you get to eat and then you cut down on the amount of calories you take in. Pretty cool right? That is like a very wonderful idea. I get to eat whatever I want for some time. Later I cut down on the intake of calories. And the best news is that I get to lose weight. Intermittent fasting has been around for a while and research has shown that it comes with a lot of health benefits. Getting really interesting? Apart from losing weight, it also comes with a lot of health benefits

· **It reduces your urge to get hungry while dieting.** For someone looking to start dieting, you definitely know that controlling that hunger urge is a massive work to accomplish. But after a few days of starting the Intermittent fasting, your body adjusts to this new eating pattern.

• **It increases your mental focus and concentration.** As you indulge in fasting, your body releases chemical called catecholamines which significantly increase your mental awareness and your productivity.

• **It stabilizes your energy levels and improves your mood.** With fewer meals, your blood sugar levels will be kept stable. This will lead to constant energy levels and help you avoid diabetes in the long run.

• **Reduced oxidative stress.**This simply means that as you fast, it reduces the accumulation of oxidative radicals in the body. This will greatly reduce damage to harm caused to internal orgas in your body.

• **It increases your capacity to resist stress, disease and aging.**Intermittent fasting, just like exercising, induces a cellular stress response in your body which increases your capacity to cope with stress and resist disease and aging.

• **You get to burn fat.** Obviously this is the main reason. You get to lose excess weight. When you eat, your body uses up the glycogen from the food you just ate to give you energy. But as you fast, your body switches to the stored fats and uses them for energy.

• **It saves you time and money.** Eating fewer meals means preparing and buying fewer meals. Hence you save money and time. Also, you are less exposed to flavours and are therefore less likely to get bored and eat something you should not.

Chapter Five

Five intermittent fasting mistakes that undo all the good work

Intermittent fasting is a general term for various eating patterns that involve not eating for short periods of time. Unlike a typical weight-loss diet that restricts how much or what you eat, intermittent fasting isn't all about the food you put in your body; instead it's about when you put that food in your body. The diet (if you can call it that) integrates periods of fasting into your day to reap the many proven benefits, like burning stored body fat for energy. It's the way we ate as hunter-gatherers, when food was scarce and we would follow feast with hours or even days of fasting. As such, intermittent fasting puts our bodies in line with the way they evolved. For me, dropping from three meals a day to two has made a vast difference to my health, and left me convinced that intermittent fasting is the missing link in our lives. However, I appreciate some people come into difficulty when trying the regime, which asks you to fast for around 16 hours in a 24 hour cycle.

Here are the top five errors people make – and how to overcome them...

1. You think it's an excuse to eat rubbish

Unfortunately, people think that intermittent fasting is a magic pill that will solve all their problems. Yes, it is an incredibly effective tool to take control of your health, but it won't cancel out eating a diet full of processed foods and sugar. When you are intermittent fasting, it is important to nourish your body with nutrient dense, whole foods. The fasting process sees your body break down damaged components and use them for energy – a cleaning, healing, slimming process. It also means your body becomes more sensitive to the food you eat; great if it's full of nourishing nutrients, not so good if you're eating crap. Not only that, if you aren't nourishing yourself with nutrient dense foods, you will feel hungry all the time.

2. You calorie restrict during your "eating window"

One of the main issues that some people come into when they start IF is that they continue to calorie restrict when they have broken their fast. The whole point of eating in this way is to listen to your body and eat until you feel full. Your body is an amazing machine, if you allow it to do its job properly. It will release hormones to make you feel full when it knows it's had enough food. If you calorie restrict you'll probably end up under-eating, which causes lots of unwanted changes in the body. Long term, it's neither sustainable nor particularly good for you.

3. You over train

If you have spent a number of years eating badly and not exercising and you would like to try IF, don't bite off more than you can chew.

Ease yourself into fasting and training gradually. One of the worst things you can do is throw yourself into a five-times-a-week intense training regime, when your body is already coming to terms with a different rhythm to your food intake. The combination can easily lead to adrenal fatigue, which will probably lay you low in bed for a week. Your body thrives with a little bit of physical stress here and there, but too much stress can become a problem. So, one thing at a time.

4. You obsess over timings and "eating windows"

In my opinion, one of the main benefits of IF is teaching you to become completely in tune with your body and understand what I call "real hunger" – something that occurs every 16-24 hours, not every 4 hours. Your body should dictate when you should eat, not the clock. If you focus on time periods, you end up counting down the hours until you can eat – you never learn to understand your body's signals.

With the two meal day, you choose to skip either breakfast or dinner, which almost automatically extends your overnight fast to about 16 hours. The focus is not on the time period; if you choose to skip breakfast you can break your fast whenever you feel hungry.

5. You aren't drinking enough water

When your body is in the fasted state it starts to break down damaged components and detoxify the body. It is very important that you flush out those toxins drinking lots of water. Ideally, you will drink more water than you usually would. I drink roughly 4-5litres every day, most of that during my fasting period. Not only that, drinking water, particularly sparling water can help you to feel full, which is important when you are first getting into IF.

Chapter Six

Using Intermittent Fasting As Help For Permanent Weight Loss

If you've been looking for a way to lose and keep weight off permanently, then you would do well to consider using intermittent fasting as a method of reducing your caloric intake to aid you in your weight loss quest.

Intermittent fasting is defined as short-term fasts, typically 24-36 hours in length, once or twice per week. These fasts are normally water only. Doing a so-called "juice fast" can defeat the purpose of intermittent fasting altogether, as by its very definition you are consuming large amounts of natural sugars, which can throw off your blood sugar as well as other bodily functions as well. Other types of fasts that emphasize one food or drink (other than water) can be just as worrisome. Short-term fasts like these are simple to do and they also provide a way to cut your caloric intake rather easily. Imagine knocking off two full days worth of calories from what you've been taking into your body. It makes the task of reducing that much easier. Of course, replacing those saved calories with massive amounts of food on the other days will negate this aid, but in truth, if you are in tune with what your body is telling you this will not be an issue. Many times we succumb to our mind's indoctrination that we'll somehow starve if we don't get that extra food. Nothing could be further from the truth.

We can survive and indeed thrive on much less food than we've been conditioned to think we need. America, in particular, is notorious when it comes to conspicuous consumption, and if we're not careful, we'll feed our next generation into an early grave with the amount of food we're forcing down their throats. There is no relief or help in sight from either the food industry, government or health organizations. Many are either trying to sell us what they have to offer, the latest diet solution (that won't work!) or deny there's a problem in the first place. (The FDA comes to mind!) So when push comes to shove the only real way to lose unwanted fat and pounds is to consume less food than we use in calories. It's simple math, and the proof that different types of diets don't matter as much as they'd like you to believe lies in the fact that most of these diets will help you to lose weight. It's being able to sustain that particular diet that becomes the problem. Most are so restrictive that it's next to impossible to do them long-term. Fasting offers a good alternative, as it's not asking you to add anything, buy anything or do anything apart from abstaining from food for a designated period of time so your body can get into calorie deficit and begin to cleanse itself. You owe it to yourself to look into this further and see if intermittent fasting might be a good idea to add to your weight loss plan.

The Lean gains fast (16/8 hour fast)

This approach was created by personal trainer Mark Berkhan and is popular among weight-lifters. The approach includes a 16 hour fast

accompany with an 8 hour feeding window. The 8 hour eating window should be the same every day. Meal frequency is not important as long as you eat during the 8 hours. The Leangains fast is done daily as opposed to once a week. This approach is highly specific and was design for weigh-lifters thus it is recommended for athletes.

Who is the approach for?

The LeanGains fast is for athletes and any serious weight lifter. It is not recommended for casual exercisers or beginners due to its complex planning.

Rules

1. Diet should be high in protein

2. You should include fasted training (training while fasted)

3. You should cycle carbohydrates (training days should be high in carbohydrates while off-days are lower in carbohydrates).

4. Feeding windows need to be consistent.

5. On training days your post workout meal should be your largest meal.

6. On non-training days your first meal should be your largest meal.

7. Be sure to take some BCAA (branch chain amino acids) before you train to ensure that you do not experience muscle loss during your fasted training.

Instructions

1. Determine your 16 hour fast period. Ideally you would want the fast to extend over night as you sleep. If you place your 16 hour fast during the time that you are awake then it would mean that your 8 hour feeding window occurs during the time you sleep. For example if your last meal is at 6:00pm on Tuesday than you would fast until

10:00am on Wednesday. Your feeding window would be from 10:00am to 6:00pm.

2. Once you decided on a fasting period your feeding window will be the remaining 8 hours of the day

3. Determine a time for training. Ideally you would want your training period to be just before you feeding window such that your first meal of the day will also be your post-training meal.

What not to do

- Do not schedule your fasting period such that your feeding window will be the same time as the time you normally sleep.

- Do not forget to take your BCAAs before you proceed with fasted-training. Most protein supplements contain BCAAs.

Below is an example of my adaptation of the Leangains program.

- Note that my training sessions are also part of the fast.

- Notice how I adapt my schedule on the weekend due to limitations such as cafeteria hours.

	Mon	Tue	Wed	Thu r	Fri	Sat	Sun
6:00 am	Trai ning	Fast ing peri od	Trai ning	Fast ing peri	Trai ning	Fast ed peri	Fast ed peri
7:00 am	sessi on		sessi on	od	sessi on	od	od

8:00 am	Feeding Window	Feeding Window	Feeding Window	Feeding Window	Feeding Window		
9:00 am							
10:00 am							
11:00 am							
12:00 am							
1:00 pm						Feeding Window	Feeding Window
2:00 pm							
3:00 pm							
4:00 pm	Fasting	Fasting	Fasting	Fasting			

5:00 pm	peri od	peri od	peri od	peri od			
6:00 pm							
7:00 pm					Fast ing peri od	Fast ing peri od	Fast ing peri od
8:00 pm							

The Warrior Diet (20/4 hour fast)

The warrior diet is a 20 hour fast period followed by a 4 hour feeding window. Like Leangains, The Warrior diet is daily too. The warrior diet was created by Ori Hofmekler and is inspired by nutritional habits of Greek warriors and Spartans. With this plan you would either fast or eat miniscule amounts of food for 18-20 hours. Then you would consume a majority of your daily caloric intake in the remaining 4-6 hours. Ideally you should place your feeding window near the end of the day as it is more convenient for family dinners and after-work training sessions. The only problem with The Warrior Diet is that trying to fit your daily caloric intake in one meal can be difficult. In summary The Warrior diet is primarily a 20 hour fast followed by one large meal. For more information check out Ori's book The Warrior Diet.

Who is this approach for?

The warrior diet is for people who are looking for an entry point into fasting. This diet is very flexible and not as strict as Leangains.

This diet is a favorite for people who love to splurge in calorie dense food (i.e. pizza, hamburgers, cakes, etc.)The warrior diet is a great introductory diet to fasting. It makes transitioning to a traditional fast easier as it allows you to have small snacks during the day given that your snacks have to consist of fruit and vegetables. If you are looking to try out fasting or get an idea of what fasting is about start with The Warrior Diet.

Rules

1. Fast for 36 hours.

2. Eat normally during the 12 hour feeding window

3. You may eat anything you like, calorie dense food in moderation of course

(unless you are severely behind on your calories and need a boost).

Instructions

1. Determine the time for your 12 hour feeding window. Note most people choose the start time as the time when they first get out of bed.

2. Your fasted period will be the remaining 12 hours of that day plus the next day. You will eat the day after your fasted day.

3. Decide if you want to eat snacks or do a complete fast during the day. Remember your snacks have to be either fruits or vegetables and maybe a protein shake.

What not to do

1. Do not eat anything calorie dense for snacks such as chips, sweets, pastries. Only fruits and vegetables are allowed (baby carrots, spinach wraps, grapes, apples, etc).

2. Do not have any large meals outside of you feeding window

3. Do not constantly switch up your one large meal (i.e. going from dinner on one day to breakfast of the next day) keep it consistent.

Example (warrior diet: dinner)

	Mon
7:00am to 5:00pm (assumes 7:00am is the start of the day)	Fasted period
6:00pm to 10:pm	Feeding Window (mainly Dinner)

The Alternate Day Fast (36/12 hours fast)

On this program you eat every other day. Basically you eat in a 12 hour window, say 7:00am to 7:00pm on Monday. Then you fast for the remainder of Monday and all throughout Tuesday. On Wednesday you eat again from 7:00am to 7:00pm. Rinse and repeat. During your feeding window you may eat anything you desire however it is recommended that you diet mainly consist of nutritional food. The alternate fast diet was popularized by Dr. James B. Johnson, please support him and buy his book, The Alternate Day Diet, if you wish to know more.

Who is this approach for?

The alternate day diet is suited for the general public i.e. the casual dieter. It is easy to pick up and apply. I would recommend this IF program for beginners as it isn't too strict and it does not have to be used in conjunction with a training program.

Rules

1. Fast for 36 hours.

2. Eat normally during the 12 hour feeding window

3. You may eat anything you like, calorie dense food in moderation of course (unless you are severely behind on your calories and need a boost).

Instructions

1. Determine the time for your 12 hour feeding window. Note most people choose the start time as the time when they first get out of bed.

2. Your fasted period will be the remaining 12 hours of that day plus the next day. You will eat the day after your fasted day.

Example (alternate day fast)

	Mon	Tue	Wed	Thu	Fri	Sat	Sun
8:0 oam to 8:0 opm	Feeding window	Fasted Period	Feeding Window	Fasted Period	Feeding window	Fasted Period	Feeding Window
The rest of the day	Fasted Period	Fasted Period	Fasted ed Period	Fasted Period	Fasted ed Period	Fasted Period	Fasted ed Period

How Can You Apply Intermittent Fasting to Your Life

Losing weight is something that a lot of people all over the world are facing the problems of. But what most people fail to realise is that intermittent fasting is the best approach that you can use to really help you lose weight when you are struggling to get those pounds lost. Losing weight is and should not have to have hard. People make a big deal out of something that should be a slow and enjoyable process that everyone can enjoy.

Intermittent fasting and fasting in general is known throughout the world something that is very good for the health. But people in general do not want to go anywhere near it. People find that fasting is something that people will struggle with but the great thing about intermittent fasting is that you only do it on occasion. Plus a day doing fasting every one in a while is a great way to get past that that plateau that you may have hit with losing the excess weight that you have on you. The best way that you can apply intermittent fasting to your life is to start slowly, and gradually increase the time that you do it. This way you will allow your body to get used to the whole process and you will see the results without having to overwhelm yourself. So the key is to start slow and slowly increase the amount of time that you do it.

Make sure that you do not do it more than once a week for maximum benefits.

Another thing that you need to take into consideration is that intermittent fasting is not the only thing that you are going to have to do to effectively lose weight. This has to be part of a big program that you are going to use in order to live a more healthy existence. You need to make sure that you diet is perfect, and you need to make sure that you are implementing a proper exercise routine into your life. Only when these things are perfect are you going to find that you will be seeing the long term results that you are after. Intermittent fasting is not an end to itself, but something that must be a part of a bigger strategy. This is the only way you are going to be successful.

Chapter Seven

Intermittent Fasting And You

Deciding if intermittent fasting is for you

Intermittent fasting isn't for everyone. Some people lose weight better on a traditional diet with regular meal frequency and some people respond better to an IF program. So before you start any IF program I recommend you try to fast for one whole day. Yep, just try not to eat anything for 24 hours. You may find out that you get irritated easily when fasting and decide that fasting is not for you. You may also discover that you are extra productive when you don't have to worry about eating and decide that you want to try out an advance IF program. So to test the waters you should

1. Fast for one full day. If your last meal is at 8:00pm on Monday try not to eat until 8.00pm on Tuesday.

Be sure to make a note of how you felt during the day. Record things like your mood, hunger, productivity and anything you deem relevant.

I want to try Intermittent Fasting

Alright so you did a 24 hour fast and decide that you would like to continue with intermittent fasting. So where do you start? The easiest way is to select one of the programs in chapter 2 and start from there.

1. Review the programs in chapter 2 and decide which one is best suited for your lifestyle

2. Follow the instructions listed with the program.

3. Keep the fast going until you reach your desired bodyweight. Note that you can keep the fast going indefinitely or end it whenever you want.

4. Be sure to record your progress and adjust accordingly.

Designing your own IF program

Alternatively if you don't like any of the programs in chapter 2 you can make your own. However I don't recommend trying this until you have some experience with IF. But if you do decide that you want to build your own program here are some steps to guide you.

First notice that all the IF programs have a few things in common. Use these commonalities as a general guideline when designing your own IF program.

- They all contain a fasted period and a feeding window

- The fasting period is generally longer than the feeding window

- Try not to have your fasting period exceed 36 hours because once it does you will start to lose the benefits of fasting and may experience actually starvation.

So if you wanted to design your own IF program.

1. First decide how often you want to fast (daily, once a week, every other day).

2. Then decide how long you want your fast period to be (36 hours maximum)

3. Then your feeding window will automatically be the remaining hours that you aren't fasting.

4. Put your plan to action the next day or the next week.

Tips for Success

Here are a few tips to keep in mind while you try out IF.

1. **Start out slow.** Take your time and slowly settle into your IF program.

Remember you don't have to maintain rigid adherence. You may want to try fasting once a month before you try fasting weekly or daily.

2. **Experiment.** Everyone is different and a cookie cutter program won't work for everyone. Start with one of the templates and adjust it to accommodate you. For example you may find out that certain foods don't agree with your bowels or you may discover that you respond better to a longer fast.

    a. a. Make a hypothesis

    b. Test it out

    c. c. Document your results

    d. Adjust

3. **Discover.** Going back to tip 3 you will discover a lot about your body. You will find things such as

- The best time for you to eat

- The easiest digestible food for your body

- The best time for you to train

- Your caloric maintenance

Once you have enough experience you won't ever fear gaining weight again as you'll know that losing it isn't as hard as everyone made it out to be.

4. **Don't fix what isn't broken.** It the diet is working and you are seeing results than leave it alone. However if fat loss has reach a plateau than consider adjusting. You may need to

lower the calories a little more (100 calories less is a good increment).

5. **Expect failure.** This tip is true for much more than just diets. The truth is very few people will succeed on their first try but what really matters is what you do afterwards. If you tried IF and didn't make any results than review what went wrong and correct it. But don't quit after one week. Give it at least one month.

6. **Listen to your body.** Our bodies are always communicating with us. It's just that most people don't know how to interpret the messages. Some common cues are listed in the following table.

Positive Cues	Negative Cues
more energy	Less energy
Better sleep	quality Less sleep
Positive mood changes (e.g. happy, relaxed, calm, less frustration	Negative mood changes (e.g. easily irritable, frustrated, anger,
Increased focus	headaches
Healthier appearance	Lack of attention

7. **Food choices are important.** Remember what I said in chapter 1 about natural foods? If not go back and reread "All are foods equal?"

8. **The best weight loss is slowest.**

People often become frustrated with diet programs because they aren't seeing immediate results. However dieting is a marathon and the best weight loss program is the one in which you lose weight in a slow consistent manner. Consider the following scenarios

> Scenario 1: person A has been dieting for 2 weeks with a severe calorie deficit. Person A has loss 10lbs in 2 weeks but now weight loss has come to a halt. Okay, so that person has managed to lose 10lbs but how much of that weight was muscle? And more

importantly will that person regain all the weight they lost?

Scenario 2: person B has been dieting for 2 weeks and has managed to lose one pound per week. However the person continues this trend for the next year and loses a total of 52lbs total with minimal muscle loss.

To sum it up strive to be in scenario 2. Record your weight weekly and make sure you lose 1 to 2 pounds a week.

9. **Be Productive.** The fast is the best time to be productive and get things done. If you are constantly focused on work then the fast would be over before you know it. However if you sit

around and brood about food, chances are you will break you fast prematurely.

10. **IF is just another component of your life.**

This is the most important tip of all of them. IF like exercise is just something we incorporate in our life to make life easier and more enjoyable. IF makes our life simpler by removing our worries about eating and allows us more time to work on other aspects of our life. If intermittent fasting causes you stress than stop doing it. In life we already have enough sources of stress you don't need another one. Remember you don't have to maintain strict adherence to an intermittent fasting program the core of intermittent fasting is, sometimes you eat, and sometimes you don't. If you can at least follow that than you will be practicing intermittent fasting in its humblest form.

Conclusion

How would you like: better control over your hunger, an easy way to lose fat and build lean attractive muscle, increased insulin sensitivity, reduced inflammation, increased growth hormone, a super efficient way of eliminating toxins, the freedom of being able to eat whatever you want without any guilt?

If I had to sum up intermittent fasting in a few rules I would say this

1. Eat sometimes but not all the time

2. When you do eat, pick the most nutritious foods

3. Indulge in your favorite foods every now and then

4. Remember to exercise.

5. "Smile, breathe, and go slowly." –

Thich Nhat HanH

References

1. Berardi, J. M., Scott-Dixon, K., & Green, N. (2012).Experiments with intermittent fasting. Precision Nutrition. Retrieved from

http://www.precisionnutrition.com/intermittent-fasting

2. Romaniello, J. (2010). Intermittent fasting 101. Retrieved from

http://www.romanfitnesssystems.com/blog/intermittent-fasting-101/

3. Romaniello, J. (2012). Intermittent fasting 201. Retrieved

from

http://www.romanfitnesssystems.com/blog/

intermittent-fasting-201/

4. Berkhan, M. (2010, April 14). The leangains guide. Retrieved from http://www.leangains.com/2010/04/leangains-guide.html

5. Park, M. (2010, Nov 08). Twinkie diet helps nutrition professor lose 27 pounds. Retrieved

from

http://www.cnn.com/2010/HEALTH/11/08/twinkie.diet.professor/index. html

6. Freediet.com daily caloric calculator. (n.d.). Retrieved

from

http://www.freedieting.com/tools/calorie_c

alculator.htm

Published by WE CANT BE BEAT LLC

www.ingramcontent.com/pod-product-compliance
Lightning Source LLC
Chambersburg PA
CBHW050917260726
48660CB00001B/257